WHAT SHOULD BE DONE WITH "ORPHANED" FROZEN EMBRYOS?

Frequently Asked Questions (FAQs)
with Magisterial Answers Quoted Directly
from *Donum Vitae* and *Dignitas Personae*

Including an Important Essay Published in
The National Catholic Bioethics Quarterly:

"The Only Moral Option is Embryo Adoption"
by Rev. Glenn Breed, MSA (+)

Edited by

Dr. Alicia Thompson, DO, MPH
Dr. Elizabeth Rex, PhD, ThD (cand.)

En Route Books and Media, LLC
Saint Louis, MO

⊕*ENROUTE*
Make the time

En Route Books and Media, LLC

5705 Rhodes Avenue

St. Louis, MO 63109

Contact us at

contactus@enroutebooksandmedia.com

Cover Credit: Sebastian Mahfood using the Dome of St. Peter's

Copyright 2025 Alicia Thompson and Elizabeth Rex

ISBN-13: 979-8-88870-346-5

Library of Congress Control Number:

Available online at https://catalog.loc.gov

Table of Contents

Foreword

Dear Readers,

We hope this book will serve as a valuable resource for everyone who is deeply concerned about the ongoing confusion regarding the ethics and the morality of Assisted Reproductive Techniques (ART), specifically In Vitro Fertilization (IVF).

There has been an urgent need for an "easy-to-read-and-understand" book dedicated to presenting the clear magisterial teachings that faithfully answer the many challenging bioethical questions and concerns that are involved with the practice of IVF.

Thankfully, the Magisterium of the Catholic Church has thoroughly researched and authoritatively promulgated the ethical and moral principles that Catholics and Christians need in the Instructions *Donum Vitae* (1987) and *Dignitas Personae* (2008).

We hope and pray that this book, filled with "Frequently Asked Questions" and "Magisterial Quotes," will provide you with the faithful ethical and moral guidance that you have been seeking.

~ Soli Deo Gloria ~

Dr. Elizabeth Rex, PhD
Dr. Alicia Thompson, DO, MPH

February 22, 2025
The Feast of the Chair of St. Peter, the Apostle
38th Anniversary of the Instruction *Donum Vitae*

WHAT SHOULD BE DONE WITH "ORPHANED" FROZEN EMBRYOS?

Frequently Asked Questions (FAQs) with Magisterial Answers Quoted Directly from *Donum Vitae* and *Dignitas Personae*

1. *As far as medical assistance is concerned, should embryos be cared for in the same way as any other human being?*

   Yes. "[S]ince the embryo must be treated as a person, it must also be defended in its integrity, tended and cared for, to the extent possible, in the same way as any other human being as far as medical assistance is concerned" *(DV* I,1).

2. *Should human embryos obtained in vitro be exposed to death?*

   No. It is "*not in conformity with the moral law deliberately to expose to death human embryos obtained in vitro*" (*DV* I, 5). (*Italics* in the original).

3. *Are all embryos produced in vitro exposed to an "absurd fate" (DV I, 5) and to "a situation of injustice which in fact cannot be resolved" (DP 19)?*

   No. *Only* "those embryos which are not transferred into the body of the mother and are called 'spare' are exposed to an absurd fate" (*DV* I,5) or "a situation of injustice" (*DP*19).

4. *Are medical and "therapeutic procedures carried out on the human embryo" licit?*

   Yes. "As with all medical interventions on patients, *one must uphold as licit procedures carried out on the human embryo which respect the life and integrity of the embryo and do not involve disproportionate risks for it but are directed toward its healing, the improvement of its condition of health, or its individual survival*" (*DV* I, 3). (*Italics* in the original).

5. *Is it licit, therefore, to transfer an embryo obtained in vitro – who is a human being and a patient - into the body of the mother as a medical intervention that is directed toward the healing and the individual survival of a human embryo obtained in vitro?*

   Yes. As stated in *DV* I, 3 - and cited in the *Catechism of the Catholic Church* # 2275 - "*one must uphold as licit procedures carried out in the human embryo*" that are directed toward its healing and "*its individual survival*" (*DV* I, 3). (*Italics* in the original).

6. *Is it licit to temporarily freeze human embryos to preserve their lives?*

    No. "Cryopreservation is *incompatible with the respect owed to human embryos*: it presupposes their production in vitro; it exposes them to the serious risk of death or physical harm, since a high percentage does not survive the process of freezing and thawing; it deprives them at least temporarily of maternal reception and gestation; it places them in a situation in which they are susceptible to further offense and manipulation" (*DP* 18; cf. *DV* I,6). (*Italics* in the original.)

7. *Can parents donate their frozen human embryos to clinical experimentation?*

    No. "No objective, even though noble in itself, such as a foreseeable advantage to science, to other human beings or to society, can in any way justify experimentation on living human embryos or fetuses, whether viable or not, either inside or outside the mother's womb. The informed consent ordinarily required for clinical experimentation on adults cannot be granted by the parents" (*DV* I, 4).

8. *May parents freely choose to thaw and let their frozen unborn child(ren) die?*

    No. Parents "may not freely dispose of the physical integrity or life of the unborn child" (*DV* I. 4).

9. *Would "the gestation of human embryos in the uterus of animals, or the hypothesis or project of constructing artificial uteruses for the human embryo" (DV I, 6) be licit?*

   No. "These procedures are contrary to the human dignity proper to the embryos" (*DV* I, 6). (*Italics* in the original).

10. *Can parents give their informed consent to whatever the type of medical, surgical or other therapy needed to heal their embryonic children?*

    Yes. "Whatever the type of medical, surgical or other therapy, the free and informed consent of the parents is required, according to the deontological rules followed in the case of children" (*DV* I, 3).

11. *Does homologous in vitro fertilization share the same ethical negativity found in extra-conjugal procreation? If not, why not?*

    No. "Certainly, homologous IVF and ET fertilization is not marked by all that ethical negativity found in extra-conjugal procreation: the family and marriage continue to constitute the setting for the birth and upbringing of the children. Nevertheless, (…) *the Church remains opposed from the moral point of view to homologous in vitro fertilization*" (*DV* II, B, 5). (*Italics* in the original.)

12. *Should a child whose human conception was achieved with IVF and ET be accepted and brought up?*

Yes. "Although the manner in which human conception is achieved with IVF and ET cannot be approved, every child which comes into the world must in any case be accepted as a living gift of the divine Goodness and must be brought up with love" (*DV* II, B, 5).

13. *Should everyone, like the Good Samaritan, treat the human embryo as a neighbor?*

Yes. "In light of the truth about the gift of human life and in the light of the moral principles which flow from that truth, everyone is invited to act (…) and, like the good Samaritan, to recognize as a neighbor even the littlest among the children of men"
(*DV* Conclusion; cf. Lk 10:29-37).

14. *Does the Catholic Church see physical sterility as an opportunity for spouses to consider adoption as an important service in the life of the human person?*

Yes. "Physical sterility in fact can be for spouses the occasion for other important services in the life of the human person, for example, adoption…" (*DV* II, B, 8).

15. *Does* **Dignitas personae** *refer to abandoned cryopreserved embryos as "orphans"?*

Yes. "The majority of embryos that are not used remain 'orphans.' Their parents do not ask for them and at times all trace of their parents is lost. This is why there are thousands upon thousands of frozen embryos in almost all countries where in vitro fertilization takes place" (*DP* 18).

16. *Does* **Donum vitae** *recommend that infertile couples consider adoption, and does* **Dignitas personae** *praise the intention of prenatal adoption for frozen embryos?*

Yes. Donum vitae teaches, "*Physical sterility* in fact can be for spouses the occasion for other *important services in the life of a person, for example, adoption...*" (*DV* II, B, 8); and **Dignitas personae,** which magisterially confirms *Donum vitae* and the "principles" and "moral evaluations which it expresses," (*DP*, Introduction) further calls *the proposal of "prenatal adoption" as "praiseworthy with regard to the intention of respecting and defending human life..."* (*DP* 19). (Emphasis added.)

17. *Is "prenatal adoption" different from 1) heterologous artificial fertilization, 2) heterologous artificial insemination, and 3) surrogate motherhood?*

Yes. "*Prenatal adoption*" involves the process of legally adopting one or more frozen human embryos as one's own legally adopted child(ren) prior to being licitly transferred to the womb for implantation, gestation, and birth. Therefore, *"prenatal adoption"* is essentially different from both *"heterologous artificial fertilization and insemination"* which involve illicit "techniques used to obtain a human conception"; and *"surrogate motherhood"* which involves the illicit agreement with a woman who is paid to carry a "pregnancy with a pledge to surrender the child once it is born" (cf. *DV* II, A, 3, Note).

18. ***Should a child who is achieved with IVF be "accepted" and "brought up with love"?***

Yes. "Although the manner in which human conception is achieved with IVF and ET cannot be approved, every child who comes into the world must in any case be accepted as a living gift of the divine Goodness and must be brought up with love" (*Donum vitae*, II, B, 5).

CONCLUSIONS

1) Artificial Reproductive Techniques (ART) - and Cryopreservation - are magisterially and morally illicit technological interventions that are prohibited.

2) However, Embryo Transfer and Prenatal Adoption are magisterially and morally licit because they are therapeutic medical procedures and interventions that heal and save the lives of "orphaned" embryos.

What Should be Done
with "Orphaned" Frozen Embryos?

- Both Instructions *condemn all forms of Artificial Reproductive Techniques (ART)*.

- Both Instructions *condemn the freezing of human embryos* (cryopreservation) because "it exposes them to the serious risk of death" and because it deprives them – even temporarily – of "maternal reception and gestation" (*DP* 18 *and DV* I, 6).

- Both Instructions *magisterially defend* the licit use of therapeutic procedures to heal and save the lives of human embryos (*DV* I, 3; and confirmed in *DP* Introduction).

- Both Instructions *magisterially praise* couples who adopt (*DV* II, B, 8; and *DP* 19).

Congregation for the Doctrine of the Faith

**Instruction *Donum vitae* on Respect for Human Life in
Its Origin and on the Dignity of Procreation:
Replies to Certain Questions of the Day
February 22, 1987**

Frequently Asked Questions About

Donum vitae

with Magisterial Answers

The following **highlighted terms and definitions** are quoted directly from the Instruction *Donum vitae.*

Introduction

1. What is the *gift of life*?

    "The gift of life which God the Creator and Father has entrusted to man calls him to appreciate the inestimable value of what he has been given and to take responsibility for it: this fundamental principle must be placed at the center of one's reflection in order to clarify and solve the moral problems raised by artificial interventions on life as it originates and on the processes of procreation." (*DV* intro. 1)

2. What are the principal *criteria* and *moral judgments* that are used in the Instruction?

    "These criteria are the respect, defense and promotion of man, his 'primary and fundamental right to life,' his dignity as a person who is endowed with a spiritual soul and with moral responsibility (*DH,* 2) and who is called to beatific communion with God." (*DV* intro., 1)

3. What are the *fundamental criteria of the moral law*?

    "Thus, science and technology require, for their own intrinsic meaning, an unconditional respect for the fundamental criteria of the moral law: that is to say, they must be at the service of the human person, of his unalienable rights and his true integral good according to the design and will of God" (*GS,* 35) (*DV* intro., 2)

4. Why is *human life sacred?*

    "Human life is sacred because from its beginning it involves 'the creative action of God' and it remains forever in a special relationship with the Creator, who is its sole end" (*DV* intro., 5)

I. Respect for Human Embryos

5. How are the terms *human generation, human being,* and *person* related?

    "Thus, the fruit of human generation, from the first moment of its existence, that is to say from the moment the zygote has formed, demands the unconditional respect that is morally due to the human being. The human being is to be respected and treated as a person from the moment of conception, and therefore from that same moment his rights as a person must be recognized, among which in the first place is the inviolable right of every innocent human being to life." (*DV* I, 1)

6. Is *prenatal diagnosis* morally licit?

    "If prenatal diagnosis respects the life and integrity oof the embryo and the human fetus and is directed towards its safeguarding or healing as an individual, then the answer is affirmative" (...) But this diagnosis is gravely opposed to the moral law when it is done with the thought of possibly inducing an abortion..." (*DV* I, 2).

7. Are *therapeutic procedures* carried out on the human embryo *licit*?

    "As with all medical interventions on patients, *one must uphold as* licit procedures carried out on the human embryo which respect the life *and integrity of the embryo and do not involve disproportionate risks for it but are directed toward its healing, the improvement of its condition of health, or its individual survival"* (DV I, 3). (*Italics* in the original for emphasis.)

8. How is one morally to evaluate research and **experimentation on human embryos** and fetuses?

"If embryos are living, whether viable or not, they must be respected just like any other person: experimentation on embryos which is not directly therapeutic is illicit" (DV I, 4). (*Italics* in the original for emphasis.)

9. Can **parents** donate their frozen human embryos to **clinical experimentation**?

"No objective, even though noble in itself, such as a foreseeable advantage to science, to other human beings or to society, can in any way justify experimentation on living human embryos or fetuses, whether viable or not, either inside or outside the mother's womb. The informed consent ordinarily required for clinical experimentation on adults cannot be granted by the parents…" (*DV* I,4).

10. May **parents** freely **dispose** (i.e., thaw, discard, etc.) of their frozen human embryos?

Parents "may not freely dispose of the physical integrity or life of the unborn child" (*DV* I,4).

11. How should the **corpses of embryos** or fetuses be treated?

"The corpses of human embryos and fetuses, whether they have been deliberately aborted or not, must be respected just as the remains of other human beings" (*DV* I,4) (*Italics* in the original for emphasis.)

12. How is one to evaluate morally the use for **research purposes** of embryos obtained by fertilization '*in vitro*'?

"It is immoral to produce human embryos destined to be exploited as disposable 'biological material'. (…) It is a duty to condemn the particular gravity of the voluntary destruction of human embryos obtained 'in vitro' for the sole purpose of research, *either by means of artificial insemination or by means of 'twin fission'"* (*DV* I, 5). (*Italics* in the original for emphasis.)

13. What judgments should be made on **other procedures** including: **twin fission, cloning, parthenogenesis, and chromosomic or genetic manipulations**?

"[A]ttempts or hypotheses for obtaining a human being without any connection with sexuality through 'twin fission,' cloning or parthenogenesis are to be considered contrary to the moral law, since they are in opposition to the dignity both of human procreation and of the conjugal union."

"Certain attempts to influence chromosomic or genetic inheritance are not therapeutic but are aimed at producing human

*beings selected according to sex or other predetermined quali-
ties. These manipulations are contrary to the personal dignity
of the human being and his or her integrity and identity"* (DV
I, 6.). (*Italics* in the original for emphasis.)

14. Is the ***freezing of embryos - cryopreservation*** - morally licit?

"*The freezing of embryos,* even when carried out in order to
preserve the life of an embryo – *cryopreservation* – *constitutes an offense against the respect due to human beings* by
exposing them to grave risks of death or harm to their physical integrity and depriving them, at least temporarily, of maternal shelter and gestation*, thus placing them in a situation
in which further offenses and manipulations are possible"
(*DV* I, 6). (*Italics* in the original.) (cf. *DP* 18)

*N.B. "*eos privet saltem ad tempus materna receptione ac ges-
tatione*" (AAS)

II. Interventions Upon Human Procreation

15. How does *Donum vitae* define **artificial procreation** or **artificial fertilization**?

"By artificial procreation or artificial fertilization are understood here the different technical procedures directed toward obtaining a human conception in a manner other than the sexual union of a man and woman." (*DV* II)

16. How does the instruction *Donum vitae* define artificial procreation or fertilization, namely, **in vitro fertilization** and **artificial insemination**?

"This instruction deals with fertilization of an ovum in a test tube (in vitro fertilization) and artificial insemination through the transfer into the woman's genital tracts of previously collected sperm." (*DV* II)

A. Heterologous Artificial Fertilization

17. What is **artificial heterologous fertilization**?

"By the term *heterologous artificial fertilization* or *procreation*, the Instruction means techniques used to obtain a human conception artificially by the use of gametes coming from at least one donor other than the spouses who are joined in marriage" (DV II, Note)

18. Should every human being always **be accepted as a gift and blessing of God**?

    "*Every human being is always to be accepted as a gift and blessing of God. However, from the moral point of view a truly responsible procreation vis-à-vis the unborn child must be the fruit of marriage*" (*DV* II, A, 1).

19. With regards to the **spouses**, *why must human procreation take place in marriage*?

    "*The fidelity of the spouses in the unity of marriage involves reciprocal respect of their right to become a father or a mother only through each other*" (*DV* II, A, 1). (Italics in original)

20. With regards to the **child**, *why must human procreation take place in marriage*?

    "The child has the right to be conceived, carried in the womb, brought into the world and brought up within marriage" (*DV* II, A, 1).

21. What is **"surrogate" motherhood**?

    By "surrogate mother "the Instruction means
    a) the woman who carries in pregnancy an embryo implanted in her uterus and who is genetically a stranger to the embryo because it has been obtained through the union of the gametes of the

'donors'. She carries the pregnancy with the pledge to surrender the baby once it is born to the party who commissioned or made the agreement for the pregnancy.

b) the woman who carries in pregnancy an embryo to whose procreation she has contributed the donation of her own ovum, fertilized through insemination with the sperm of a man other than her husband. She carries the pregnancy with a pledge to surrender the child once it is born to the party who commissioned or made the agreement for the pregnancy" (*DV* II, 3, Note).

22. Is "surrogate" motherhood morally licit?

"No, for the same reasons which lead one to reject heterologous artificial fertilization: for it is contrary to the unity of marriage and to the dignity of the procreation of the human person. (*DV* II, 3).

B. Homologous Artificial Fertilization

23. What is **homologous artificial fertilization**?

"By artificial *homologous fertilization* or *procreation*, the Instruction means the technique used to obtain a human conception using the gametes of the two spouses joined in marriage. (DV II, Note)

24. Can a child be desired or conceived as *the product of an intervention of medical or biological techniques*?

"He cannot be desired or conceived as the product of an intervention of medical or biological techniques; that would be the equivalent to reducing him to an object of scientific technology." (*DV* II, B, 4 c.)

25. Do researchers who transfer some embryos and not others *usurp the place of God*?

"By acting in this way the researcher usurps the place of God; and even though he may be unaware of this, het set himself up as the master and of the destiny of others inasmuch as he arbitrarily chooses whom he will allow to live and whom he will send to death, and kills defenseless human beings" (*DV* I, 5).

26. Should human embryos obtained *in vitro* be *deliberately exposed to death*?

It is "not in conformity with the moral law deliberately to expose to death human embryos obtained in vitro" (*DV* I, 5).

27. What happens to the *embryos which are not transferred into the body of the mother*?

"In consequence of the fact that they have been produced *in vitro*, those embryos which are not transferred into the body of the mother and are called "spare" are exposed to an absurd fate, with no possibility of their being offered safe means of survival which can be pursued" (*DV* I, 5).

28. Is homologous IVF and ET brought about by the actions of ***third parties***?

"Homologous IVF and ET is brought about outside the bodies of the couple through actions of third parties whose competence and technical activity determine the success of the procedure." (*DV* II, B, 5).

29. Does homologous IVF and ET fertilization establish a ***relationship of domination***?

"Such fertilization entrusts the life and identity of the embryo into the power of doctors and biologists and establishes the domination of technology over the origin and destiny of the human person. Such a relationship of domination is in itself contrary to the dignity and equality that must be common to parents and children" (DV II, B, 5).

30. Is homologous IVF and ET fertilization marked with the same ***ethical negativity*** found in [heterologous] extra-conjugal procreation?

"Certainly, homologous IVF and ET fertilization is not marked by all that ethical negativity found in [heterologous] extra-conjugal procreation; *the family and marriage continue to constitute the setting for the birth and upbring of the children.* Nevertheless, in conformity with the traditional doctrine relating to the goods of marriage and the dignity of the person, the Church remains opposed from the moral point of view to homologous *in vitro* fertilization" (DV II, B, 5). (*Italics* added for emphasis)

31. Should an embryo conceived by IVF and ET be **accepted as a living gift**?

"Although the manner in which human conception is achieved with IVF and ET cannot be approved, every child which comes into the world must in any case be accepted as a living gift of the Divine Goodness and must be brought up with love."
(DV II, B, 5)

III. Moral and Civil Law

32. How does legislation regulate the relationships between *civil law* and *moral law*?

"The intervention of the public authority must be inspired by the rational principles which regulate the relationships between civil law and moral law. The task of civil law is to ensure the common good of people through the recognition of and the defense of fundamental rights and through the promotion of peace and public morality" (*DV* III; cf. *Dignitatis humanae, 7*).

33. Do *inalienable human rights of the person* depend on *parents*, *society*, or the *state*?

"[T]he inalienable rights of the person must be recognized and respected by civil society and the political authority. These human rights depend neither on single individuals nor on parents; nor do they represent a concession made by society and the state: they pertain to human nature and are inherent in the person by virtue of the creative act from which the person took his or her origin" (*DV* III).

34. What *fundamental rights* must be recognized and respected by civil society?

"Among such fundamental rights one should mention in this regard:

a) every human being's right to life and physical integrity from the moment of conception until death.

b) the rights of the family and of marriage as an institution and, in this area, the child's right to be conceived, brought into the world, and brought up by his parents" (*DV* III).

Conclusion

35. Does *Donum vitae* refer to embryos as **neighbors** and as *the least of our brethren*?

"In the light of the truth about the gift of human life and in the light of the moral principles which flow from that truth, everyone is invited to act in the area of responsibility proper to each and, like the Good Samaritan, to recognize as a neighbor even the littlest among the children of men (cf. *Lk* 10:29-37). Here Christ's words find a new and particular echo: "What you do to one of the least of my brethren, you do unto me" (*Mt* 25:40). (*DV*, Conclusion)

Congregation for the Doctrine of the Faith

Instruction *Dignitas personae*
on Certain Bioethical Questions
September 8, 2008

Frequently Asked Questions About

Dignitas personae

with Magisterial Answers

The following **highlighted terms and definitions** are quoted directly from the Instruction *Dignitas personae*:

Introduction

1. What is meant by the ***"dignity of a person"?***

   "The dignity of a person must be recognized in every human being from conception to natural death. This fundamental principle expresses a great "yes" to human life and must be at the center of ethical reflection on biomedical research, which has as greater importance in today's world" (*DP* Intro).

2. What is the *spirit of the Hippocratic Oath* that is mentioned in *Dignitas personae*?

    "In the current multifaceted philosophical and scientific context, a considerable number of scientists and philosophers, in the spirit of the Hippocratic Oath, see in medical science a service to human fragility aimed at the cure of disease, the relief of suffering and the equitable extension of necessary care to all people" (*DP* 2).

3. How does the Catholic Church evaluate *biomedical research on human life*?

    "In presenting principles and moral evaluations regarding biomedical research on human life, the Catholic Church draws upon the light of both reason and of faith and seeks to set forth an integral vision of man and his vocation..." (*DP* 3).

Part I: Anthropological, Theological, and Ethical Aspects of Human Life and Procreation

4. What is the *fundamental ethical criterion* in *Dignitas personae* to evaluate all moral questions that relate to procedures involving the human embryo?

    "It is appropriate to recall the fundamental ethical criterion in the Instruction *Donum vitae* in order to evaluate all moral questions that relate to procedures involving the human embryo: 'Thus, the fruit of generation, from the first moment of its existence, that is to say, from the moment the zygote has formed, demands the unconditional respect that is morally due to the human being in his bodily and spiritual totality. The human being is to be respected and treated as a person from the moment of conception; and therefore from that same moment his rights as a person must be recognized, among which in the first place is the inviolable right of every innocent human being to life'" (*DP* 4; cf. *DV*, I, 1).

5. What is the ***anthropological and ethical status*** and ***the dignity*** of the human embryo?

    "'[H]ow could a human individual not be a human person?' (*DV* I,1) Indeed, the reality of the human being for the entire span of life, both before and after birth, does not allow us to posit either a change in nature or a gradation in moral value, since it possesses full anthropological and ethical status. The human embryo has, therefore, from the very beginning, the dignity proper to a person" (*DP* 5).

6. Where is ***the authentic context of the origin of human life***?

    "Marriage, present in all times and in all cultures, 'is in reality something wisely and providentially instituted by God the Creator with a view to carrying out his loving plan in human beings.' (…) *The origin of human life has its authentic context in marriage and the family,* where it is generated through an act which expresses the reciprocal love between a man and a woman. Procreation which is truly responsible vis-s-vis the child to be born 'must be the fruit of marriage'" (*DP* 6; cf. *HV* 8; cf., *DV* II, A, 1). (*Italics* in the original.)

7. Does the *mystery of man* become clear through the *mystery of the Incarnation*?

"In the mystery of the Incarnation, the Son of God confirmed the dignity of the body and soul which constitute the human being. Christ did not disdain human bodiliness, but instead disclosed its meaning and value: 'in reality, it is only in the mystery of the incarnate Word that the mystery of man truly becomes clear'" (*DP* 7; cf. *GS* 22).

8. Must all *discrimination with regard to human dignity* be excluded?

"The introduction of discrimination with regard to human dignity based on biological, psychological, or educational development, or based on health-related criteria, must be excluded. At every stage of his existence, man, created in the image and likeness of God, reflects 'the face of his only begotten Son…. This boundless and almost incomprehensible love of God for the human being reveals the degree to which the human person deserves to be loved in himself, independently of any other consideration…'" (*DP* 8; cf. Benedict

XVI in "The Human Embryo in the Pre-implantation Phase;" in 2008 AAS 98, 264).

9. Are the natural and supernatural acts of procreation a *reflection of trinitarian love*?

"These two dimensions of life, the natural and supernatural, allow us to understand better the sense in which the acts that permit a new human being to come into existence, in which a man and a woman give themselves to each other, are a reflection of trinitarian love. 'God, who is love and life, has inscribed in man and woman the vocation to share in a special way in his mystery of personal communion and in his work as Creator and Father'" (*DP* 9; cf. *DV*, Introduction, 3).

10. How does the Catholic Church gauge the *ethical value of biomedical science*?

"The Catholic Church gauges the ethical value of biomedical science in reference to both *the unconditional respect owed to every human being at every moment of his or her existence, and the defense of the specific character of the personal act which transmits life.* The intervention of the Magisterium falls within the mission of contributing to the formation of conscience, by authentically teaching the truth which is Christ and at the same time by declaring and confirming authoritatively the principles of the moral order which spring from human nature itself" (*DP* 10).

Second Part: New Problems Concerning Procreation

11. Are there **new questions and problems** concerning procreation since *Donum vitae*?

    "In light of the principles recalled above, certain questions regarding procreation which have emerged and have become more clear in the years since the publication of *Donum vitae* can now be examined" (*DP* 11).

Techniques for Assisting Fertility

12. What **fundamental goods** must be respected regarding the **treatment of infertility**?

13. "With regard to the treatment of infertility, new medical techniques must respect three fundamental goods:

    a) The right to life and to physical integrity of every human being from conception to natural death;

    b) The unity of marriage, which means reciprocal respect for the right within marriage to become father or mother only together with the other spouse;

    c) The specifically human values of sexuality which require 'that the procreation of a human person be brought about as the fruit of the conjugal act specific to the love between spouses.' (*DP* 12)

"In light of this principle, all techniques of heterologous artificial fertilization, as well as those techniques of homologous artificial fertilization which substitute the conjugal act are to be excluded" (*DP* 12).

"The doctor is at the service of the persons and of human procreation. He does not have the authority to dispose of them or to decide their fate" (*DP* 12).

"Homologous artificial insemination within marriage cannot be admitted except for those cases in which technical means is not a substitute for the conjugal act but serves to facilitate and to help so that the act attains its natural purpose" (*DP* 12).

13.1 Are *techniques aimed at removing obstacles to natural fertilization licit?*

"Certainly, techniques aimed at removing obstacles to natural fertilization, as do for example, hormonal treatments for infertility, surgery for endometriosis, unblocking fallopian tubes or their surgical repair, are licit. (…) None of these treatments replaces the conjugal act, which alone is worthy of truly responsible procreation" (*DP* 13).

13.2 Should **adoption** be encouraged, promoted and facilitated by legislation?

"In order to come to the aid of the many infertile couples who want to have children, adoption should be encouraged, promoted and facilitated by appropriate legislation so that many children who lack parents may receive a home that will contribute to their human development" (*DP* 13).

13.3 Should research and investment be directed at **the prevention of sterility**?

"In addition, research and investment directed at the prevention of sterility deserve encouragement" (*DP* 13).

In vitro Fertilization and the Deliberate Destruction of Embryos

14. Does the process of *in vitro* fertilization involve the **deliberate destruction of embryos**?

"The fact that the process of *in vitro* fertilization very frequently involves the deliberate destruction of embryos was already noted in the Instruction *Donum vitae*. Subsequent experience has shown, however, that all techniques of *in vitro* fertilization proceed as if the human embryo were simply a mass of cells to be used, selected, and discarded." (*DP* 14)

"These losses are accepted by the practitioners of *in vitro* fertilization as the price to be paid for positive results (…) but does not manifest a concrete interest in the right to life of each individual embryo" (*DP* 14)

15. What are some of the cases where **the destruction of embryos is willed and foreseen**?

"It is true that not all the losses of embryos in the process of *in vitro* fertilization have the same relationship to the will of those involved in the procedure. But it is also true that in many cases the abandonment, destruction and loss of embryos are foreseen and willed" (*DP* 15).

"Embryos produced *in vitro* which have defects are directly discarded" (*DP* 15).

"Cases are becoming ever more prevalent in which couples who have no fertility problems are using artificial means of procreation in order to engage in genetic selection of their offspring" (*DP* 15)

"It is now common to stimulate ovulation so as to obtain a large number of oocytes which are then fertilized. Of these, some are transferred into the woman's uterus, while the others are frozen for future use" (*DP* 15).

"The practice of multiple embryo transfer implies a purely utilitarian treatment of embryos. (…) In fact, techniques of in vitro fertilization are accepted based on the presupposition that the individual embryo is not deserving of full respect in the presence of the competing desire for offspring, which must be satisfied" (*DP* 15).

"This sad reality, which often goes unmentioned, is truly deplorable: the 'various techniques of artificial reproduction, which would seem to be at the service of life and which are frequently used with this intention, actually open the door to new threats against life"
(*DP* 15; cf. *EV* 14)

16. Is it *ethically unacceptable to disassociate procreation from the conjugal act*? **Is the life of every human embryo in its pre-implantation stage sacred and inviolable?**

"The Church moreover holds that is ethically unacceptable to *disassociate procreation from the integrally personal context of the conjugal act*: human procreation is a personal act of a husband and a wife, which is not capable of substitution" (*DP* 16) (*Italics* in the original.)

"The blithe acceptance of the enormous number of abortions involved in in the process of in vitro fertilization vividly illustrates how the replacement of the conjugal act by a technical procedure – in addition to being in contradiction with the respect that is due to procreation as something that cannot be reduced to mere reproduction – leads to the weakening of the respect owed to every human being. (*DP* 16)

"Such a desire [for a child] cannot justify the 'production' of offspring, just as the desire not to have a child cannot justify the abandonment or destruction of a child once he or she has been conceived" (*DP* 16)

"Therefore, the Magisterium of the Church has constantly proclaimed the sacred and inviolable character of every human life from its conception until its natural death" (*DP* 16; cf. Benedict XVI in "The Human Embryo in the Pre-implantation Phase;" in 2008 AAS 98, 264).

Intracytoplasmic Sperm Injection (ICSI)

17. Is *Intracytoplasmic Sperm Injection (ICSI) intrinsically illicit*?

"This technique is used with increasing frequency given its effectiveness in overcoming various forms of male infertility. Just as in general with *in vitro* fertilization, of which it is a variety, ICSI is intrinsically illicit" (*DP* 17).

Freezing Embryos

18. Why is **cryopreservation incompatible** with the respect owed to human embryos? And why are **abandoned frozen embryos called "orphans" in Dignitas personae**?

"Cryopreservation is incompatible with the respect owed to human embryos: it presupposes their production in vitro; it exposes them to the serious risk of death or physical harm, since a high percentage does not survive the process of freezing and thawing; it deprives them at least temporarily of maternal reception and gestation; it places them in a situation in which they are susceptible to further offense and manipulation" (*DP* 18; cf. *DV* I, 6).

"The majority of embryos that are not used remain "orphans". Their parents do not ask for them and at times all trace of the parents is lost. This is why there are thousands upon thousands of frozen embryos in almost all countries where *in vitro* fertilization takes place" (*DP* 18).

19. What does *Dignitas personae* teach regarding the question of **what to do with the large number of frozen embryos already in existence**?

"With regard to *the large number of frozen embryos already in existence* the question becomes: what to do with them?" (*DP* 19)

"Proposals *to use these embryos for research or for treatment of disease* are obviously unacceptable because they treat the embryos as mere 'biological material' and result in their destruction" (*DP* 19).

"The proposal that these embryos could be put at the disposal of infertile couples as a *treatment for infertility* is not ethically acceptable for the same reasons which make artificial heterologous procreation illicit as well as any form of surrogate motherhood; this procedure would also lead to other problems of a medical, psychological and legal nature" (*DP* 19).

"It has also been proposed, soley in order to allow human beings to be born who are otherwise condemned to destruction, that there could be a form of *'prenatal adoption'*. This proposal, praiseworthy with regard to the intention of respecting and defending human life, presents however various problems not dissimilar to those mentioned above" (*DP* 19).

"All things considered it needs to be recognized that the thousands of abandoned embryos represent *a situation of injustice which in fact cannot be resolved*" (*DP* 19).

"Therefore John Paul II made an appeal to the conscience of the world's scientific authorities and in particular to doctors, that the production of human embryos be halted, taking into account that there seems to be no morally licit solution regarding the human destiny of the thousands and thousands of 'frozen' embryos which are and remain the subjects of essential rights and should therefore be protected by law as human persons" (*DP* 19; cf. John Paul II, "*Evangelium vitae* and the Law" in AAS 88 in 1996, 943-944).

The Freezing of Oocytes

20. Is the *freezing of oocytes for the purpose of procreation morally acceptable*?

"[I]t needs to be stated that cryopreservation of oocytes for the purpose of being used in artificial procreation is to be considered morally unacceptable" (*DP* 20).

Reduction of Embryos

21. *Is the deliberate and intentional elimination of an embryo an intentional abortion*?

"From the ethical point of view, *embryo reduction is an intentional selective abortion*. It is in fact the deliberate and direct elimination of one or more innocent human beings in the initial phase of their existence and as such always constitutes a grave moral disorder" (*DP* 21). (*Italics* in the original.)

"At other times, moral principles are invoked, such as those of the lesser evil or double effect, which are likewise inapplicable in this case. It is never permitted to do something which is intrinsically illicit, not even, in view of a good result: *the end does not justify the means*" (*DP* 21). (*Italics* in the original.)

Preimplantation Diagnosis

22. Does *preimplantation diagnosis express a eugenic mentality* and *when does it constitute an act of abortion*?

"Preimplantation diagnosis is form of prenatal diagnosis connected to techniques of artificial fertilization in which embryos formed *in vitro* undergo genetic diagnosis before being transferred into the woman's womb. Such diagnosis is done *in order to ensure that only embryos free from defects or having the desired sex or other particular qualities are transferred*" (*DP* 22). (*Italics* in the original.)

"Preimplantation diagnosis - connected as it is with artificial fertilization, which is always intrinsically illicit – is directed toward the *qualitative selection and consequent destruction of embryos*, which constitutes an act of abortion" (*DP* 22).

"Preimplantation diagnosis is therefore the expression of a *eugenic mentality* that 'accepts selective abortion in order to prevent the birth of children affected by various types of anomalies. Such an attitude is shameful and utterly reprehensible, since it presumes to measure the value of a human life only within the parameters of "normality" and physical well-being, thus opening the way to legitimizing infanticide and euthanasia as well'" (*DP* 22; cf. *EV* 63).

New Forms of Interception and Contragestation

23. Are technical means of "*interception*" and "*contragestation*" that prevent or interfere with implantation (after fertilization) generally considered to be abortifacients?

"Alongside methods of preventing pregnancy [...] there are other technical means which act after fertilization, when the embryo is already constituted, either before or after implantation in the uterine wall. Such methods are interceptive if they interfere with the embryo before implantation and contragestative of the cause the elimination of the embryo once implanted" (*DP* 23).

"It must be noted that, however, that anyone who seeks to prevent the implantation of an embryo which may possibly have been conceived and who either requests or prescribes such a pharmaceutical, generally intends abortion" (*DP* 23).

Third Part: New Treatments Which Involve the Manipulation of the Embryo or the Human Genetic Patrimony

24. What is *regenerative medicine* and the *treatment of genetically based diseases*?

    "Knowledge acquired in recent years has opened new perspectives for both regenerative medicine and for the treatment of genetically based diseases" (*DP* 24).

Gene Therapy

25. What is *gene therapy,* which is commonly called *techniques of genetic engineering*?

    "*Gene therapy* commonly refers to techniques of genetic engineering applied to human beings for therapeutic purposes, that is to say, with the aim of curing genetically based diseases" (*DP* 25).

26. Is *somatic cell therapy* morally licit? Is *germ line cell therapy* morally illicit?

    "*Procedures used on somatic cells for strictly therapeutic purposes are in principle morally licit.* (...) The informed consent of the patient or his legitimate representative is also required" (*DP* 26). (*Italics* in the original.)

"The moral evaluation of *germ line cell therapy* is different. Because the risks connected to any genetic manipulation are considerable and as yet not fully controllable, *in the present state of research, it is not permissible to act in a way that may cause possible harm to the resulting progeny*" (*DP* 26). (*Italics* in the original.)

"It needs to be added that this only takes place in the context of *in vitro* fertilization and thus runs up against all the ethical objections to such procedures. For these reasons, therefore, it must be stated that, in its current state, germ line cell therapy in all its forms is morally illicit" (*DP* 26).

27. Should **genetic engineering** be used for purposes **other than medical treatment**?

"*The question of using genetic engineering for purposes other than medical treatment also calls for consideration.* Some have imagined the possibility of using techniques of genetic engineering to introduce alterations with the presumed aim of improving and strengthening the gene pool" (*DV* 27).

"In stating the ethical negativity of these kinds of interventions which imply *an unjust domination of man over man,* the Church also recalls the need to return to an attitude of care for people and of education in accepting human life in its concrete finite nature" (*DP* 27). (*Italics* in the original)

Human Cloning

28. What is *human cloning*?

"Human cloning refers to the asexual or agametic reproduction of the entire human organism in order to produce one or more "copies" which, from a genetic perspective, are substantially identical to the single original" (*DP* 38).

29. Why is *human cloning illicit*?

"Human cloning is intrinsically illicit in that, by taking the ethical negativity of techniques of artificial fertilization to their extreme, it seeks to *give rise to a new human being without a connection to the act of reciprocal self-giving between the spouses* and, more radically, *without any link to sexuality*. This leads to manipulation and abuses gravely injurious to human dignity" (*DP* 29).

"The originality of every person is a consequence of the particular relationship that exists between God and a human being from the first moment of his existence and carries with it the obligation to respect the singularity and integrity of each person, even on the biological and genetic levels" (*DP* 29).

30. Why is *therapeutic cloning gravely immoral*?

"To create embryos with the intention of destroying them, even with the intention of helping the sick, is completely incompatible with human dignity. *[...] It is gravely immoral to sacrifice a human life for therapeutic ends"* (*DP* 30). (*Italics* in original.)

The Therapeutic Use of Stem Cells

31. What are **stem cells**?

"Stem cells are undifferentiated cells with two basic characteristics:

a) the prolonged capability of multiplying themselves while maintaining the undifferentiated state;

b) the capability of producing transitory progenitor cells from which fully differentiated cells descend, for example, nerve cells, muscle cell and blood cells" (*DP* 31).

32. What is the **ethical evaluation** of the **risks** and the **methods of obtaining stem cells**?

"With regards to the ethical evaluation, it is necessary to consider *the methods of obtaining stem cells as well as the risks connected with their clinical and experimental use"* (*DP* 32) (*Italics* in original.)

"The obtaining of stem cells from a living human embryo invariably causes the death of the embryo and is consequently gravely illicit" (*DP* 32).

"Research initiatives involving the use of adult stem cells, since they do not present ethical problems, should be encouraged and supported" (DP 32).

Attempts at Hybridization

33. Why is *hybrid cloning* an offense against the dignity of human beings?

"Recently animal oocytes have been used for programming the nuclei of human somatic cells – this is generally called hybrid cloning – in order to extract embryonic stem cells from the resulting embryos without having to use human oocytes" (*DP* 33).

"From the ethical standpoint, such procedures represent an offense against the dignity of human beings on account of *the admixture of human and animal genetic elements capable of disrupting the specific identity of man*" (DP 33). (*Italics* in original.)

The Use of Human "Biological Material" of Illicit Origin

34. Why are all forms of *experimentation on human embryos* always gravely immoral?

"For scientific research and for the production of vaccines or other products, cell lines are at times used which are the result of an illicit intervention against the life or physical integrity of a human being" (*DP* 34).

"'[T]he use of human embryos or fetuses as an object of experimentation constitutes a crime against their dignity as human beings who have a right to the same respect owed to a child once born, just as to every person.' These forms of experimentation always constitute a grave moral disorder" (*DP* 34; cf. *EV* 63).

35. Should researchers refuse to use "**biological material**" obtained from in vitro fertilization and abortion?

"Therefore, it needs to be said that there is a duty to refuse to use such "biological material" even when there is no close connection between the researcher and the actions of those who performed the artificial fertilization and abortion" (*DP* 35).

"This duty springs from the necessity to *remove oneself, within the area of one's own research, from a gravely unjust legal situation and to affirm with clarity the value of human life*" (*DP* 35). (*Italics* in the original.)

Conclusion

36. What has human history shown about *unjust discrimination and oppression*, and about understanding and *recognizing the value and dignity of every person*?

"Human history shows, however, how man has abused and continues to abuse power and capabilities which God has entrusted to him, giving rise to *various forms of unjust discrimination and oppression* of the weakest and most defenseless" (*DP* 36).

"At the same time, human history has also shown real *progress in the understanding and recognition of the value and dignity of every person* as the foundation of the rights and ethical imperatives by which human society has been and continues to be structured" (*DP* 36).

"Precisely in the name of promoting human dignity, therefore, practices and forms of behavior harmful to that dignity have been prohibited" (*DP* 36).

37. **Why did the Congregation of the Doctrine of the Faith write *Dignitas personae*?**

"In virtue of the Church's doctrinal and pastoral mission, the Congregation for the Doctrine of the Faith has felt obliged to reiterate both the dignity and the fundamental and inalienable rights of every human being, including those in the initial stages of their existence, and to state explicitly the need for protection and respect which this dignity requires of everyone" (*DP* 37).

"The Christian faithful will commit themselves to the energetic promotion of a new culture of life by receiving the contents of this Instruction with the religious assent of their spirit of their spirit, knowing that God always gives the grace necessary to observe his commandments and that, in every human being, above all in the least among us, one meets Christ himself" (cf. Mt 25:41). In addition, all persons of good will, in particular physicians and researchers, open to dialogue and desirous of knowing what is true, will understand and agree with these principles and judgments, which seek to safeguard the vulnerable condition of human beings in the first stages of life and to promote a more human civilization" (*DP* 37).

The Only Moral Option
Is Embryo Adoption

Br. Glenn Breed, MSA

Abstract. Approximately 800,000 human embryos are currently in cryostorage in the United States. The Catholic Church holds that in vitro fertilization (IVF) and cryopreservation of human embryos are intrinsically evil. IVF continues to increase at a rate of approximately 9 percent per annum. Many Catholic couples have used IVF as a means to conceive a child. There are typically additional embryos that are cryopreserved for later use. Once a couple has reached the number of children they desire, they are faced with a very difficult moral decision regarding the disposition of their remaining frozen embryos. The biological parents must choose one of four options. Three result in death of their frozen embryos. Only one can possibly result in life. The only moral option is embryo adoption, a life-giving choice that is strongly supported by Sacred Scripture and Sacred Tradition. *National Catholic Bioethics Quarterly* 14.3 (Autumn 2014): 441–447.

There is an extremely serious and growing problem in the United States and around the world: namely, what to do with hundreds of thousands of "leftover" frozen human embryos that are created using in vitro fertilization and then routinely cryopreserved and stored. IVF and cryopreservation are both intrinsically evil acts. "The number of babies born as a result of assisted reproduction technologies (ART) has reached an estimated total of 5 million since the world's first, Louise Brown, was born in July 1978. ... The cumulative total of births was put at 4.6 million last year, and this year

Glenn Breed, a brother in the Society of the Missionaries of the Holy Apostles, has a master's degree in Sacred Scripture and is pursuing a master's degree in divinity at Holy Apostles College and Seminary in Cromwell, Connecticut.

[2012] has now reached an approximate total of 5 million."[1] This is an increase of approximately four hundred thousand births or 8.7 percent in one year.

When the Society for Assisted Reproductive Technology (SART) released its 2012 report on assisted reproductive technologies in the United States, it reported the following statistics:

> SART's 379 member clinics performed 165,172 cycles, or procedures involv-ing IVF, in 2012. These procedures resulted in the birth of 61,740 babies, an increase of more than 2,000 infants from 2011. There were an estimated 3.9 million babies born in the US in 2012, thus IVF babies now constitute over 1.5% of all births [in the United States]. This is the largest number of cycles, of babies and percentage of babies born through IVF ever reported.[2]

The total of 61,740 babies is a very important statistic as there are normally many more embryos created and frozen than the number of births utilizing IVF. As many as twenty oocytes may be harvested, and from these, twenty embryos may be created contemporaneously. Although some of these IVF-conceived human embryos may be discarded as "biological hazardous waste," most are cryopreserved and stored for future "use."

In association with SART and the RAND Corporation, David Hoffman, MD, and colleagues reported in 2003 that the estimated number of frozen embryos at IVF clinics in the United States was nearly four hundred thousand.[3] And according to E. Christian Brugger, "that number increases annually by approximately 19,000, which puts estimates in 2010 at between 500,000 and 600,000 frozen human embryos."[4] Using 8.7 percent as a growth rate in IVF, the estimated number of frozen embryos in storage in the United States in 2013 was approximately 800,000.

Disposition of Abandoned Embryos

One of the most serious immoral consequences of IVF is an ever-increasing number of abandoned cryopreserved embryos. Let us suppose that the genetic parents have twenty embryos created through IVF; they then transfer two embryos into the mother and decide to cryopreserve the other eighteen embryos for potential use at a later time. Suppose that the parents now have a set of twin girls and are faced with a very difficult moral decision of life and death for their stored frozen embryos. They decide they have the number of children they desire and make the immoral decision to abandon their remaining cryopreserved embryos.

---

[1] European Society of Human Reproduction and Embryology, *Science Daily*, July 2, 2012, http://www.sciencedaily.com/releases/2012/07/120702134746.htm.

[2] Society for Assisted Reproductive Technology, February 17, 2014, http://www.sart.org/SART_Technology_Releases_New_Annual_Report_on_In_Vitro_Fertilization_Procedures/.

[3] David I. Hoffman et al., "Cryopreserved Embryos in the United States and Their Availability for Research," *Fertility and Sterility* 79.5 (May 2003): 1063–1069.

[4] E. Christian Brugger, "Rescuing Frozen Embryos: Is Adoption a Valid Moral Option?," *Zenit*, March 17, 2010, http://www.zenit.org/en/articles/rescuing-frozen-embryos.

One reason for this decision is the continued cost of cryopreservation. The typical storage cost to maintain cryopreserved human embryos is approximately $50 per month.[5] When the frozen embryos are abandoned, the storage company has to make a decision. Four options are possible: (1) keep the embryos frozen, (2) thaw out the embryos and discard them as biological hazardous waste, (3) give them to medical science for experimentation and ultimate destruction, or (4) make them available for adoption. Causing the direct death of a human frozen embryo is intrinsically evil regardless of the method. The solution one might reach through faith and reason is to offer married Catholic couples the cryopreserved embryos for adoption. The only life-giving, moral option is prenatal embryo adoption.

Church's Teaching on Life

The Old and New Testaments and Sacred Tradition teach us that life is precious, a gift from God, and that we are to protect the innocent. It is illicit and immoral to kill an innocent human person regardless of his or her state. The Old Testament proclaims, "Whoever sheds the blood of man, by man shall his blood be shed; for God made man in his own image" (Gen. 9:6). Each of us is made *Imago Dei* (in the image of God), and the fifth commandment of the Decalogue states unambiguously, "You shall not kill" (Exod. 20:13, Deut. 5:17).

"Man's life comes from God; it is his gift, his image and imprint, a sharing in his breath of life. God therefore is the sole Lord of this life: man cannot do with it as he wills. ... Human life and death are thus in the hands of God, in his power. ... He alone can say: 'It is I who bring both death and life' (Deut. 32:39)."[6] "Human life is sacred because from its beginning it involves the creative action of God and it remains forever in a special relationship with the Creator, who is its sole end. God alone is the Lord of life from its beginning to its end: no one can, in any circumstance, claim for himself the right to destroy directly an innocent human being."[7]

As demonstrated above, it is explicit in Sacred Scripture and Sacred Tradition that no man can take the life of another innocent human being. Who is more innocent than an abandoned, voiceless, captive, homeless, and cryopreserved human embryo? The answer is self-evident: nobody.

Human Embryo Adoption Is Good and Licit

The morality of human embryo adoption does not change, but science changes rapidly. The following is a good example. In the spring of 2001, Elio Cardinal Sgreccia, the former president of the Pontifical Academy for Life, said "that embryo adoption has 'an end which is good' and cannot be dismissed as illicit. But given the high failure rate of implantation and the fact that the process of freezing and

---

[5] FertilityProRegistry Network, "Cost and Financing of Embryo Freezing," accessed June 30, 2014, http://www.fertilityproregistry.com/article/cost-and-financing-of-embryo-freezing.html.

[6] John Paul II, *Evangelium vitae* (March 25, 1995), n. 39.

[7] *Catechism of the Catholic Church*, n. 2258, as quoted in John Paul II, *Evangelium vitae*, n. 53.

THE NATIONAL CATHOLIC BIOETHICS QUARTERLY ✢ AUTUMN 2014

thawing may cause many embryos to suffer genetic damage, he concludes, 'Can we really counsel women to do this? It would mean counseling heroism. ... The issue is one big question mark. The point is, we should never have gone down this road to begin with.'"[8]

Yes, we in the United States should not have gone down the IVF road, and IVF should be banned, but in the United States, banning IVF will be a long time coming, as there are many infertile couples who desire children. The medical technology exists, and IVF demand is increasing, which results in more cryopreserved embryos residing in storage.

The first part of Elio Cardinal Sgreccia's statement remains correct in that embryo adoption has "an end which is good and cannot be dismissed as illicit." The portion of the statement concerning rates of implantation and the process of freezing and thawing are now incorrect. Science has advanced at a very rapid rate. In 2001, it was true that in the slow freezing process, up to 50 percent of embryos had intracellular genetic damage, and the live birth rates were about 30 to 40 percent.

Using the vitrification cryopreservation process (now five years old), approximately 97 percent of the embryos frozen are recovered without intracellular genetic damage.[9] Dr. Kuwayama claims a 100 percent freezing and recovery rate using his cryotech technique.[10] In 2003, the success rate of live births per cycle for women under age 35 was 37 percent, compared with approximately 42 percent in 2009.[11] There are many factors that determine the IVF success rate of live births, and the stated success rate of 42 percent is now nearly five years old.

Since 2009, medical procedures have advanced: testing the quality of the oocyte, testing the quality of the sperm, cryopreservation of the embryo, genetic testing of the embryos, grading of embryos, growing the embryo to the blastocyst stage before transfer into the woman, hormonal preparation of the woman, and other methods used in the IVF process to increase success rates.

Some of these procedures are licit and some are illicit. As science continues to advance, the rate of success of IVF live births will increase. The more successful IVF, the more human embryos will be created and cryopreserved. Some will be abandoned and left as orphans.

---

[8] "Lives in Limbo: Embryos on the Edge of Ethics," *Zenit*, December 8, 2001, http://www.zenit.org/article-17177?l=english.

[9] Mojtaba Rezazadeh Valojerdi et al., "Vitrification versus Slow Freezing Gives Excellent Survival, Post Warming Embryo Morphology and Pregnancy Outcomes for Human Cleaved Embryos," *Journal of Assisted Reproduction and Genetics* 26.6 (June 2009): 347–354.

[10] Masashige Kuwayama, "History of Dr. Kuwayama's Vitrification Methods," YouTube video, 12:05, filmed April 28, 2012, at Cryotech India's Live, Hands-On Workshop on Vitrification of Oocytes and Embryos in Mumbai, India, posted by "CryotechIndiaVideos," August 21, 2012, https://www.youtube.com/watch?v=WkF3bBCJ12A.

[11] David Barad, "IVF Success Rates," *Center for Human Reproduction*, January 15, 2013, http://www.centerforhumanreprod.com/ivf-success-rates.html.

Adoption of Orphans Is Not New

When the biological parents make the decision to abandon their frozen embryos, they become orphans in the eyes of God, as they are fatherless and motherless. Sacred Scripture directs us to love, provide for, and protect defenseless orphans. Moses is an excellent example of adoption in a time of danger:

> Now the daughter of Pharaoh came down to bathe at the river, and her maidens walked beside the river; she saw the basket among the reeds and sent her maid to fetch it. When she opened it she saw the child; and lo, the babe was crying. She took pity on him and said, "This is one of the Hebrews' children." Then his sister said to Pharaoh's daughter, "Shall I go and call you a nurse from the Hebrew women to nurse the child for you?" And Pharaoh's daughter said to her, "Go." So the girl went and called the child's mother. And Pharaoh's daughter said to her, "Take this child away, and nurse him for me, and I will give you your wages." So the woman took the child and nursed him. And the child grew, and she brought him to Pharaoh's daughter, and he became her son; and she named him Moses, for she said, "Because I drew him out of the water. (Exod. 2:5–10)

Moses (Mosheh, משה) means "saved from the water." In the case of a frozen human embryo, they are saved from liquid nitrogen. Moses's mother gave him up for adoption to the Pharaoh's daughter; otherwise, he would have been killed. Pharaoh's daughter adopted Moses to save his life. She was his adoptive mother. Is this any different from an adoptive mother who saves the life of a frozen embryo? Whether you are in a tarred basket floating down the Nile River surrounded by crocodiles or floating in a test tube surrounded by liquid nitrogen, your life is at risk unless someone intervenes. Adoption has a long-standing tradition, as evidenced by the adoption of Moses the prophet, God's chosen one to lead his people.

The object of the act of adoptive parents is to protect a human life, be it in utero, ex utero (baby or child), a fresh human embryo, or an abandoned frozen one (orphan). The parents' choice of adoption serves to protect and nurture a human life at various stages of life. The end objective in the case of prenatal adoption is to grow and birth the child, raise the child to maturity, and be the parents till death. A wrong has been done to the orphan; the adoptive parents are doing a good for the orphan whose life is innately good and worthy of protection. The adoptive parents' only interest is to protect and give life to an abandoned, unborn, and orphaned baby.

There are many passages in the Old and New Testaments where God has proclaimed a special interest in and love for orphans and children. "Give justice to the weak and the fatherless; maintain the right of the afflicted and the destitute" (Ps. 82:3). Who is more weak, afflicted, and destitute than an abandoned cryopreserved human embryo in storage? "Thus says the Lord: Do justice and righteousness, and deliver from the hand of the oppressor him who has been robbed. And do no wrong or violence to the alien, the fatherless, and the widow, nor shed innocent blood in this place" (Jer. 22:3).

Doing violence and shedding the blood of the innocent abandoned human embryo is immoral. "For my father and my mother have forsaken me, but the Lord will take me up" (Ps. 27:10). The Lord will not forsake the orphaned frozen embryo. He will deliver justice to those who harm them. Abandoned by their parents, they become strangers and are oppressed. God hears their cry. We offend God by not

445

The National Catholic Bioethics Quarterly ✢ Autumn 2014

taking action to save them from a cruel death. It is a sin of omission to not help our brothers and sisters who are enslaved in a test tube in liquid nitrogen.

Health Care for Orphaned Frozen Embryos

Donum vitae says that "one must hold as licit procedures carried out on the human embryo which respect the life and integrity of the embryo and do not involve disproportionate risk to it, but are directed toward its healing, the improvement of its condition of health, or its individual survival." [12] So those procedures that heal, improve the health, or assist in the individual survival of the frozen embryo are licit. Embryo adoption meets the above moral and health criteria and is therefore licit, moral, and life giving. "Catholic health care ministry witnesses to the sanctity of life from the moment of conception until death." [13]

The first right of the human person, the right to life, entails "a right to the means for the proper development of life, such as adequate health care." [14] A frozen embryo is a human person, and his or her life must be defended, as he or she is precious in the eyes of God. They must be given proper health care and be assisted in their development of life. "It is not in conformity with the moral law to deliberately expose to death human embryos obtained 'in vitro.'" [15] If these frozen embryos are disposed of as biological hazardous waste, or thawed out and left to die on the counter, or given to medical science for experimentation, or simply remain in a frozen state, they are being exposed to death. There are many loving married couples available to adopt these abandoned, forsaken, and abused cryopreserved human embryos.

Corporal Works of Mercy

The corporal works of mercy (*Catechism*, n. 2447) apply to the treatment of abandoned frozen human embryos. We are called to perform these works on their behalf:

- Feed the hungry: a mother's womb is where they receive physical, emotional, and psychological gifts.
- Shelter the homeless (welcome the stranger): a mother's womb and an adoptive family become their future home.
- Clothe the naked: embryos are naked and cold; they need a mother's warmth.
- Visit the sick and imprisoned: they are sick, dying, and imprisoned.
- Bury the dead: those who are not transferred into a loving mother face a certain death alone.

---

[12] Congregation for the Doctrine of the Faith, *Donum vitae* (February 22, 1987), I.3, as quoted in the *Catechism*, n. 2275.

[13] US Conference of Catholic Bishops, *Ethical and Religious Directives for Catholic Health Care Services*, 5th ed. (Washington, DC: USCCB, 2009), part 4.

[14] John Paul II, Discourse to Those Taking Part in the Thirty-Fifth General Assembly of the World Medical Association (October 29, 1983), *AAS* 76 (1984): 390.

[15] CDF, *Donum vitae*, I.5.

Sacred Scripture encourages us to care for the needy, the poor, the sick, and the least among us. "For the poor will never cease out of the land; therefore I command you, You shall open wide your hand to your brother, to the needy and to the poor, in the land" (Deut. 15:11).

The pharaohs today are those that keep these frozen embryos enslaved by not providing them an opportunity to be free and to live. "If a brother or sister is ill-clad and in lack of daily food, and one of you says to them, 'Go in peace, be warmed and filled,' without giving them the things needed for the body, what does it profit?" (James 2:15–16). These frozen embryos are in desperate need of a mother's womb, which provides food, shelter, and clothing. They need release from slavery. They need visitation, mercy, and the care of a loving adoptive family. Currently many of them die, but they are not buried, just forgotten, except by God. God does not forget His children or those who abandon or kill them. When we encourage and act in favor of the adoption of abandoned frozen human embryos, we are performing corporal works of mercy.

"Truly, I say to you, as you did it to one of the least of these my brethren, you did it to me. Then he will say to those at his left hand, Depart from me, you cursed, into the eternal fire prepared for the devil and his angels" (Matt. 25:40–41). We are called by God to care for the least among us, and I would submit to you that the abandoned human embryos are the least among us as they are innocent, destitute, voiceless, homeless, and without hope unless we act to give them an opportunity for life.

The only moral option for an abandoned human embryo is adoption into a loving family. The abandoned embryo is a good human person without actual sin and exists as a person from the moment of conception. What he or she needs is a maternal environment in which to grow until birth and then to live life as a member of a loving family. Killing the unborn human embryo is not a viable option, as it is gravely immoral, contrary to the fifth commandment of the Decalogue, and is offensive to God. Adoption is the only moral option.

447

In Memoriam

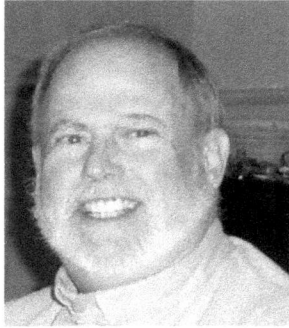

Father Glenn Breed, MSA

(https://msa-usa.org/blog/msa-news/obituary-of-father-glenn-ray-breed-msa)

September 11, 2022

Fr. Glenn Breed, 74, was born on June 27, 1948, in Cheyenne, Wyoming, and died on September 11, 2022, in Cheyenne.

Glenn Ray Breed was a geophysicist in the oil exploration business working for Texas Instruments and British Petroleum. He spent much of his career in Middle Eastern countries and was even in Iran during the beginning of the revolution in the late 1970s.

Later in life, he studied theology at Holy Apostles Seminary in Cromwell, Connecticut, and was ordained a Roman Catholic Priest on November 30, 2016. Father Glenn belonged to the Society of the Missionaries of Holy Apostles and spent the last months of his life ministering to the sick at the Cheyenne VA Hospital while also studying Bioethics and Moral Theology at Catholic University of America and in preparation for a doctoral dissertation on the morality of embryo adoption.

An Obituary Tribute
Written by Dr. Elizabeth Rex
on October 11, 2022

Dear Fr. Glenn,

You were my star student studying Catholic Bioethics at Holy Apostles College & Seminary.

I was also honored to be your advisor for a Directed Study course during which you wrote an outstanding essay titled, *"The Only Moral Option is Embryo Adoption"* that was published in *The National Catholic Bioethics Quarterly.*

You were a man and a priest who truly loved and defended the tragic lives of the very least of our brethren, millions of abandoned frozen human embryos.

Fr. Glenn fully embraced Our Lord's words, "What you do unto the least of my brethren, you do unto Me."

Thank you for all you did to courageously speak up and defend the lives of countless innocent unborn children.

Please pray for us! And may you Rest in Eternal Peace.

Your friend,

Dr. Elizabeth Rex